What Happens Next?

DEALING WITH LIFE CHANGES

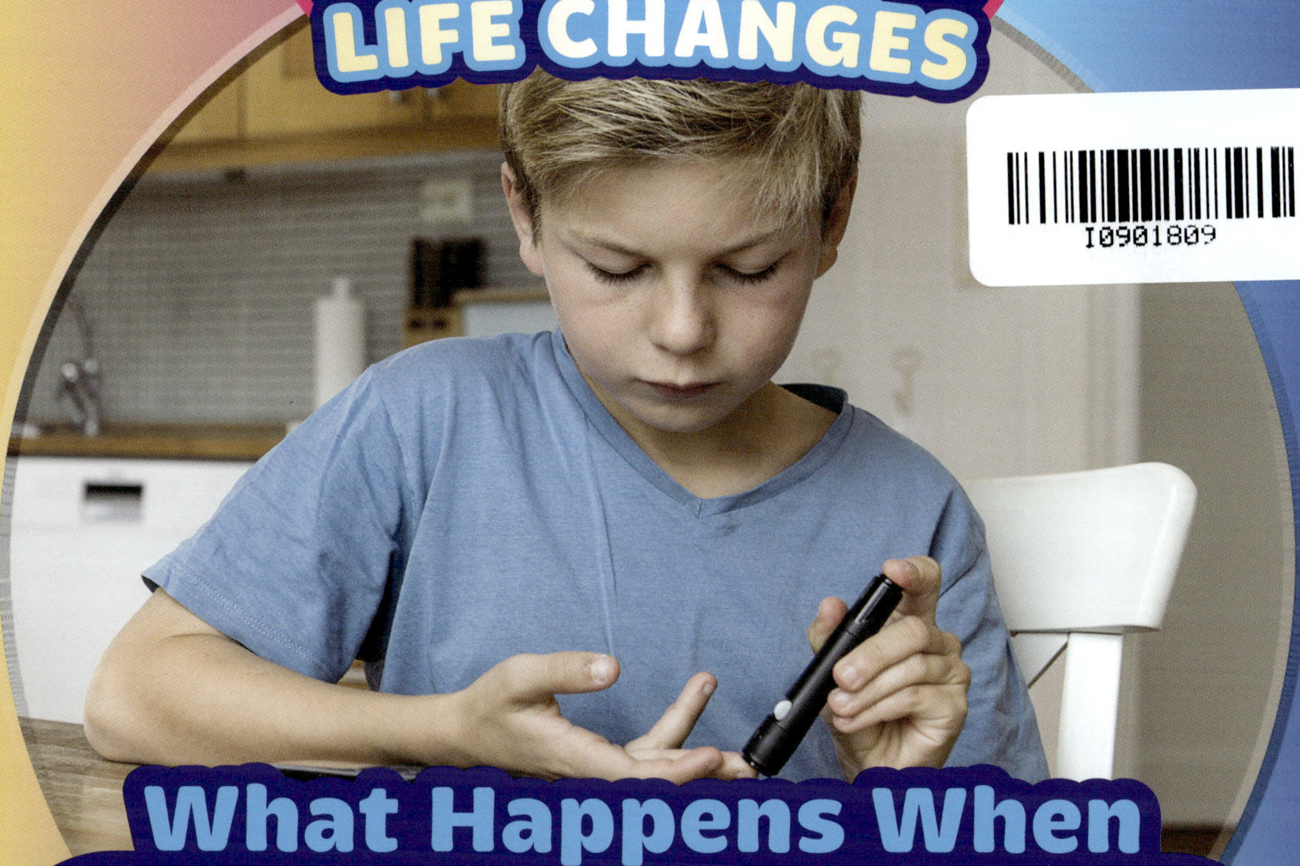

What Happens When I Have Diabetes?

Therese M. Shea

PowerKiDS press

Published in 2025 by The Rosen Publishing Group, Inc.
2544 Clinton Street, Buffalo, NY 14224

First Edition

Editor: Theresa Emminizer
Book Design: Leslie Taylor

Photo Credits: Cover R Kristoffersen/Shutterstock.com; p. 5 matimix/Shutterstock.com; p. 7 Designua/Shutterstock.com; p. 9 JPC-PROD/Shutterstock.com; p. 11 WilleeCole Photography/Shutterstock.com; p. 12 Mr Doomits/Shutterstock.com; p. 13 File:Jonge-diabetespatint-met-insulinepomp-op-de-huid-geplakt-1326488205.jpg/wikicommons.com; p. 15 Proxima Studio/ Shutterstock.com; p. 17 MillaF/Shutterstock.com; p. 19 Queenmoonlite Studio/Shutterstock.com; p. 21 mother_ana/ Shutterstock.com.

Cataloging-in-Publication Data

Names: Shea, Therese M.
Title: What happens when I have diabetes? / Therese M. Shea.
Description: Buffalo, NY : PowerKids Press, 2025. | Series: What happens next? dealing with life changes| Includes glossary and index.
Identifiers: ISBN 9781725327177 (pbk.) | ISBN 9781725327191 (library bound) | ISBN 9781725327207 (ebook)
Subjects: LCSH: Diabetes–Juvenile literature. | Diabetes in children–Juvenile literature. | Diabetes in children–Treatment–Juvenile literature. | Diabetes in children–Prevention–Juvenile literature.
Classification: LCC RC660.5 S54 2025 | DDC 618.92'462–dc23

Manufactured in the United States of America

CPSIA Compliance Information: Batch #CSPK25. For Further Information contact Rosen Publishing at 1-800-237-9932.

CONTENTS

Not Just an Illness

When you're a kid, being sick colors everything. Playdates, game nights, and even birthdays aren't as fun. Many illnesses come on quickly and go away quickly. But sometimes, the feeling of being unwell lasts longer.

For some kids, that sickness isn't a sickness. It's a condition that won't go away called diabetes. Diabetes means your body can't use a sugar in foods in the right way. This sugar, called glucose, builds up in the blood and causes problems. Luckily, diabetes can be treated.

Your Point of View

The sugar glucose is a main fuel of the body. A fuel is something used to produce energy, or power.

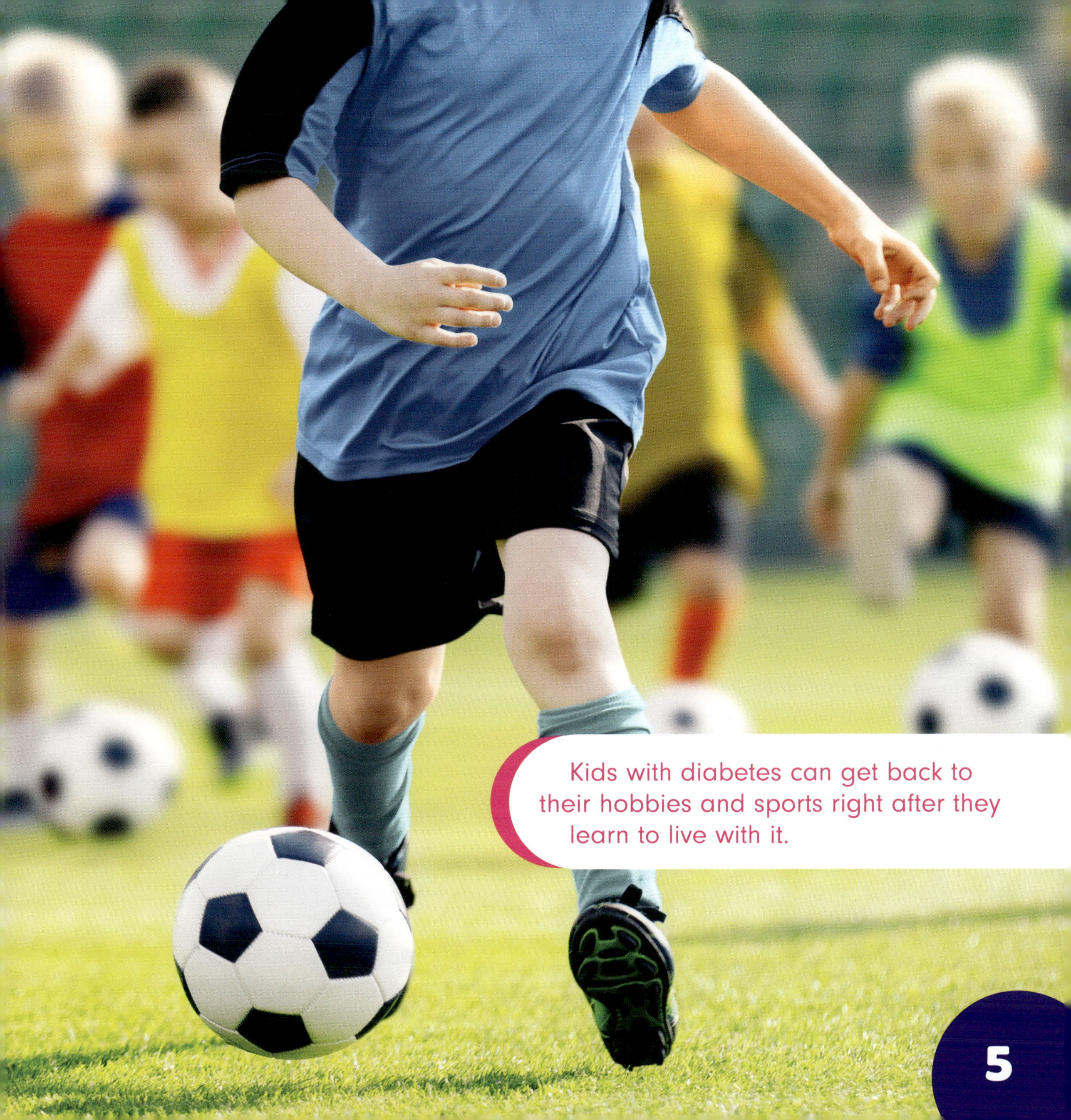

Kids with diabetes can get back to their hobbies and sports right after they learn to live with it.

What's Going Wrong?

Picture yourself eating your favorite food. Many foods have the sugar glucose. When your body digests, or breaks down, your food, it puts the glucose into your blood. At the same time, a body part called the pancreas should make the **hormone** insulin. Insulin tells the body's cells to let the glucose in. The cells use glucose to produce energy.

If you have diabetes, your pancreas is the problem. It either doesn't make insulin or doesn't make insulin that works. That leaves too much glucose in your blood.

Importance of Insulin

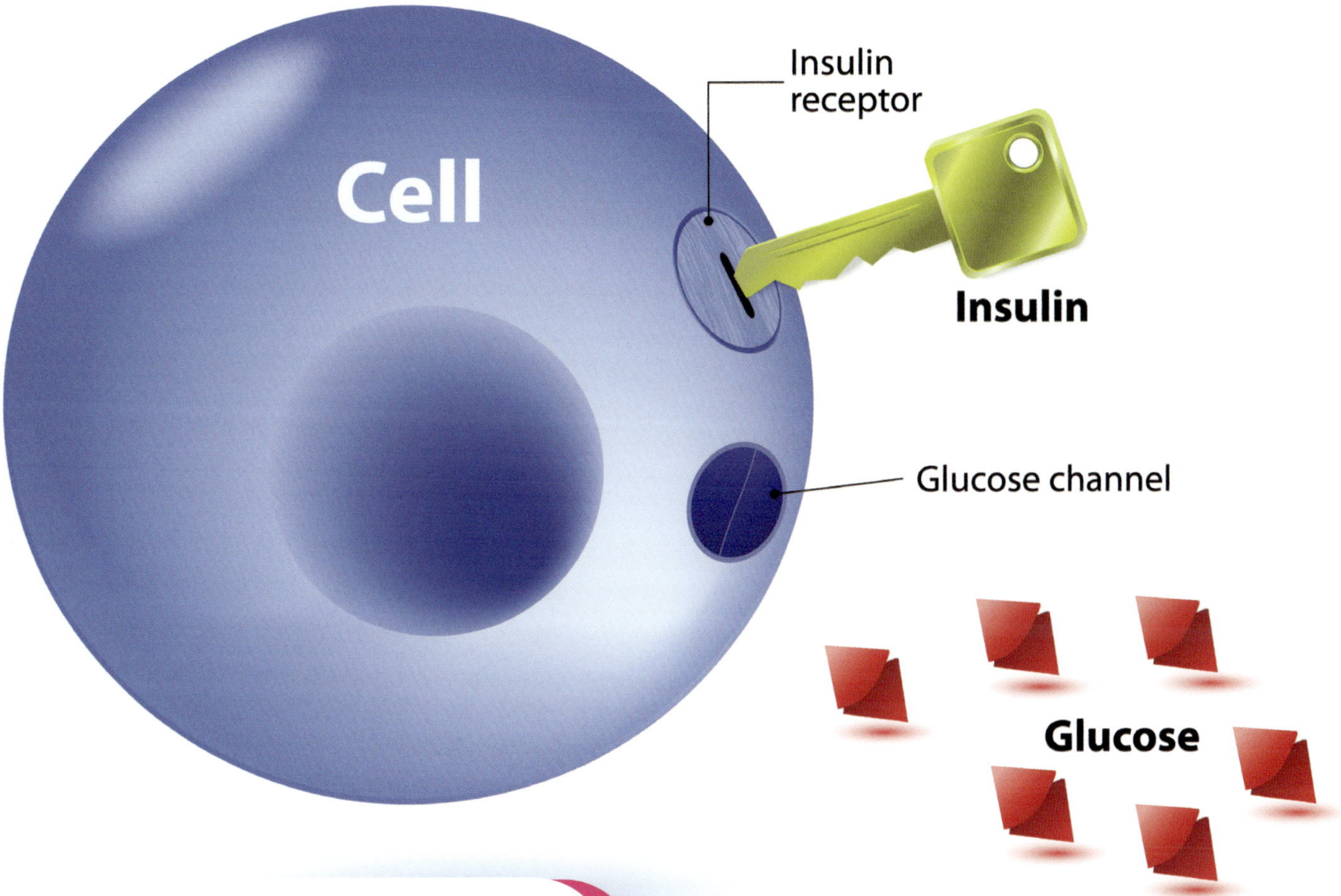

Insulin is the key to opening the cells for glucose.

Symptoms

Symptoms of diabetes can include being thirsty and hungry a lot, urinating (peeing) often, and feeling very tired. Some kids with diabetes have fuzzy eyesight and unusual weight loss.

A doctor uses blood tests to check glucose in your blood. Another blood test can tell what type, or kind, of diabetes you have. Type 1 diabetes means your pancreas isn't making insulin. Type 2 diabetes means the pancreas makes insulin that doesn't work well. It's important to know which kind of diabetes because treatment plans for each are different.

Many kids don't like blood tests. But your blood tells the story of what's going on in your body!

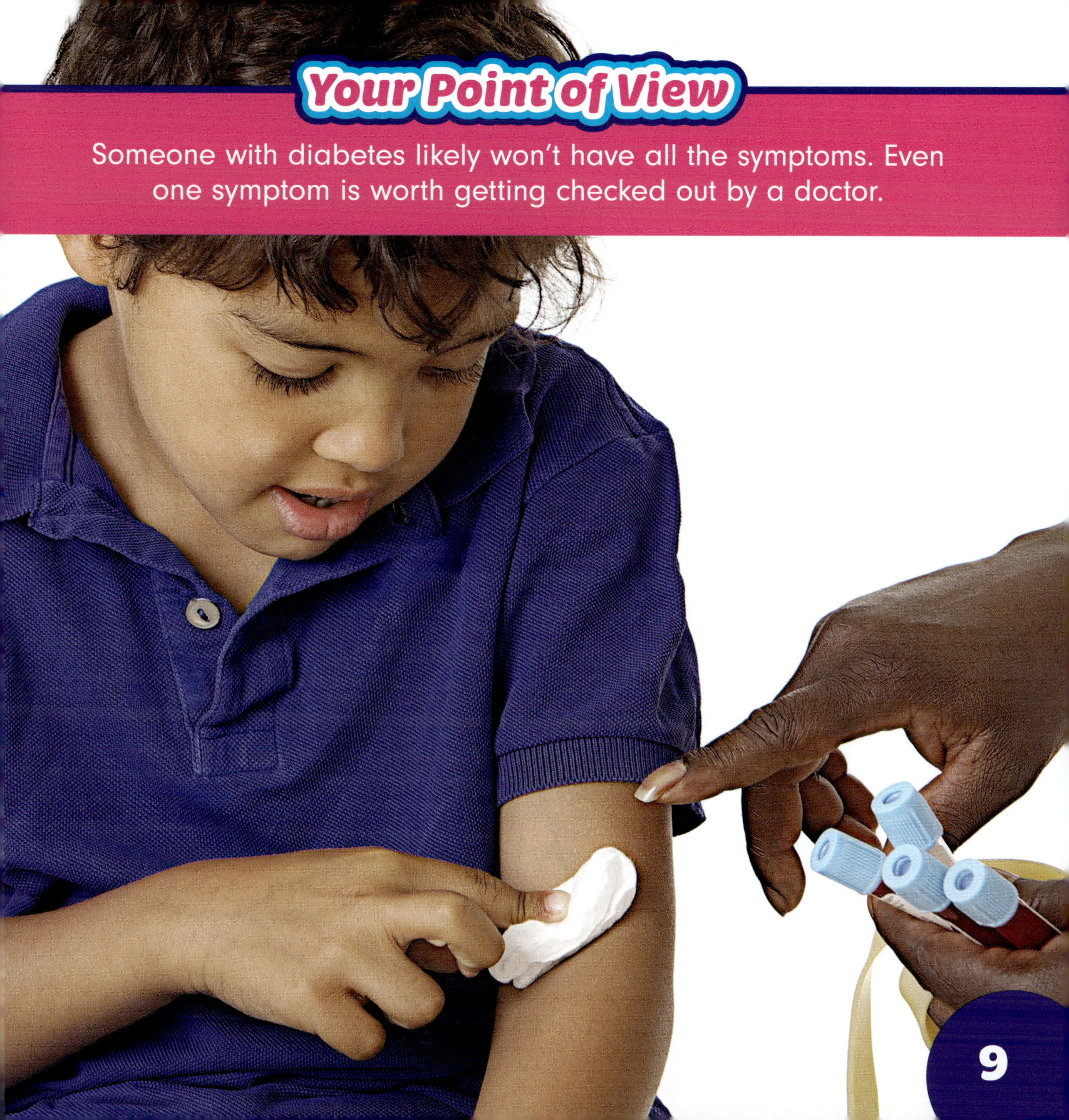

Your Point of View

Someone with diabetes likely won't have all the symptoms. Even one symptom is worth getting checked out by a doctor.

What's the Danger?

When too much glucose remains in your blood, your body lacks energy. The liver turns body fat into **acids** called ketones. Ketones enter the blood. Too many ketones are harmful to the body.

Diabetes can harm **nerves** that help you feel. Your fingers and toes may feel tingly or numb. It can harm kidneys, which clean waste from your blood. It can also hurt your **blood vessels**, causing eye and heart problems. But diabetes treatments can stop these things from happening to your body.

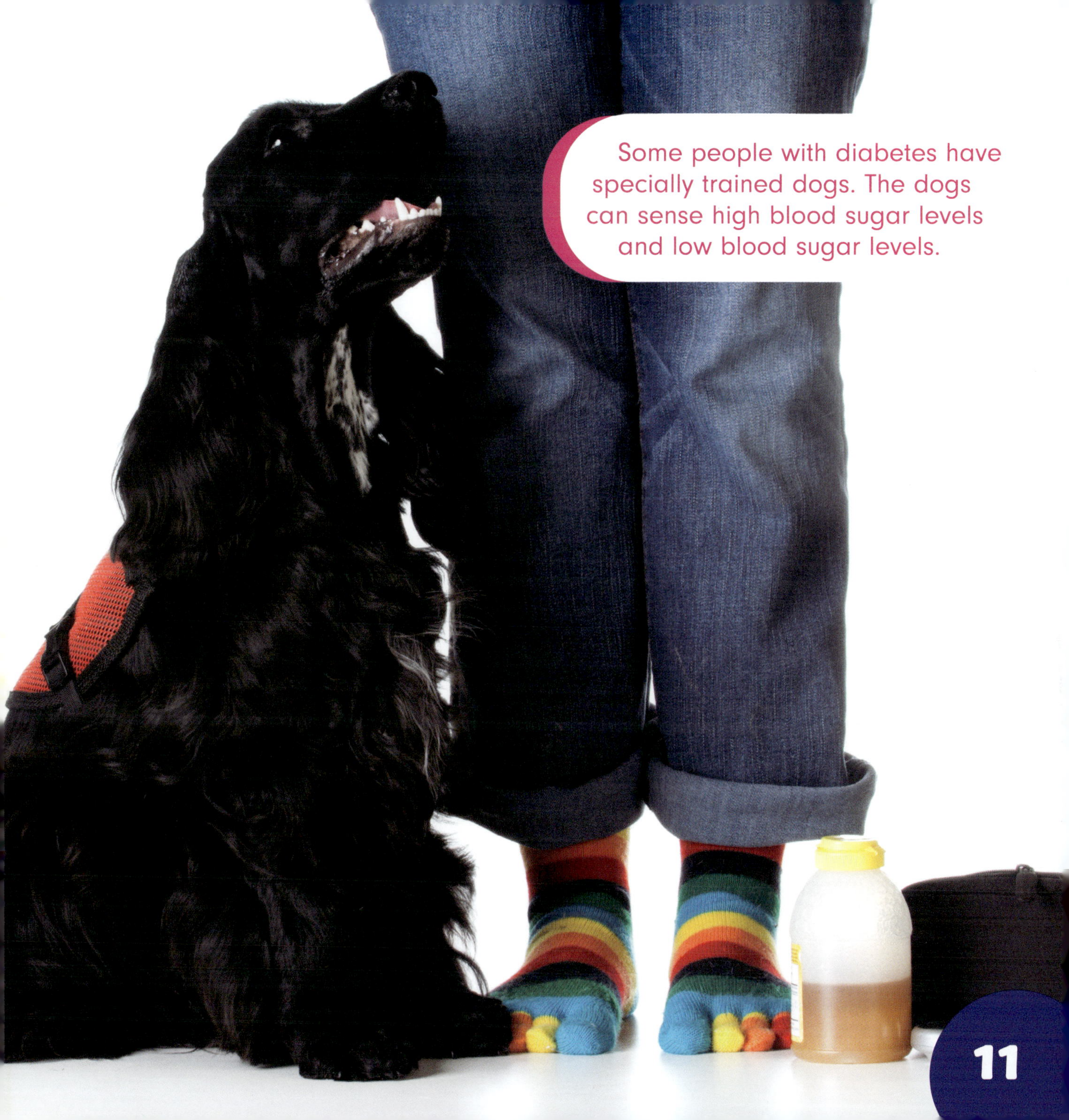

Some people with diabetes have specially trained dogs. The dogs can sense high blood sugar levels and low blood sugar levels.

Type 1 Treatment

If you have type 1 diabetes, your doctor will plan a treatment just for your body. You'll learn to monitor, or watch, your blood sugar level. It needs to stay in a certain range. You'll learn when and how to take insulin.

Two ways to take insulin are by injection, or shot, and by pump. Injections use needles. Some, called injection pens, are especially easy to use. An insulin pump is a device, or tool, you wear. It uses a tiny tube to deliver insulin into the body as needed.

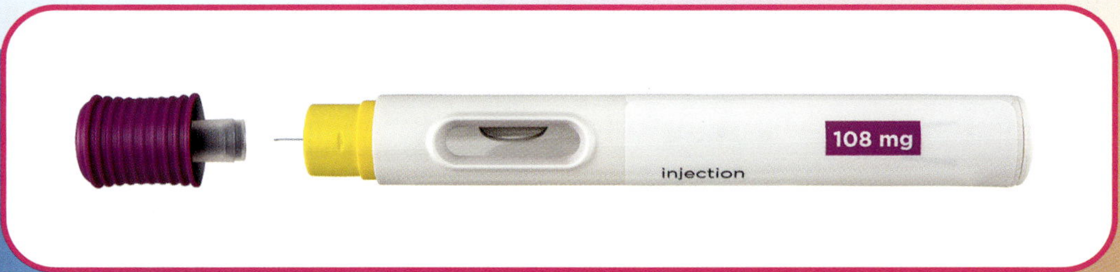

Your Point of View

Low blood sugar level, or hypoglycemia, is another danger for kids with type 1 diabetes. Taking too much insulin, not eating enough, or exercising a lot can cause it. Eating or drinking a bit of something sugary can help.

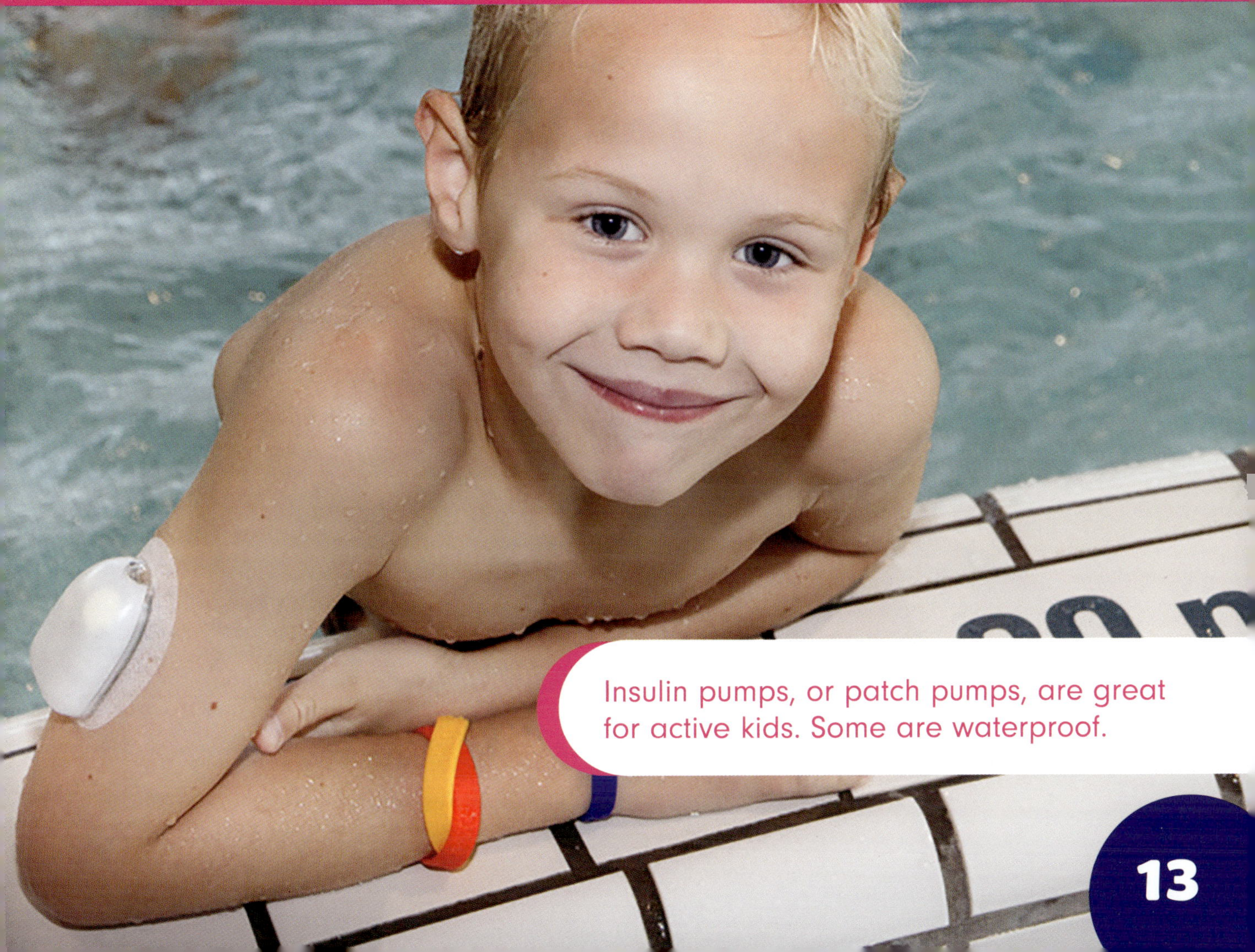

Insulin pumps, or patch pumps, are great for active kids. Some are waterproof.

Type 2 Treatment

If you have type 2 diabetes, your special treatment plan will also include checking your blood sugar levels. You may take insulin by an injection or through an insulin pump. You'll also need to eat healthy foods and exercise regularly.

Those with type 2 diabetes may be able to change their body's **reaction** to glucose through their treatment plan. It's possible to reach a point when your body no longer needs to take insulin.

Your Point of View

Some medications, or drugs, can help kids manage their diabetes. Medications might be a part of some diabetes treatment plans.

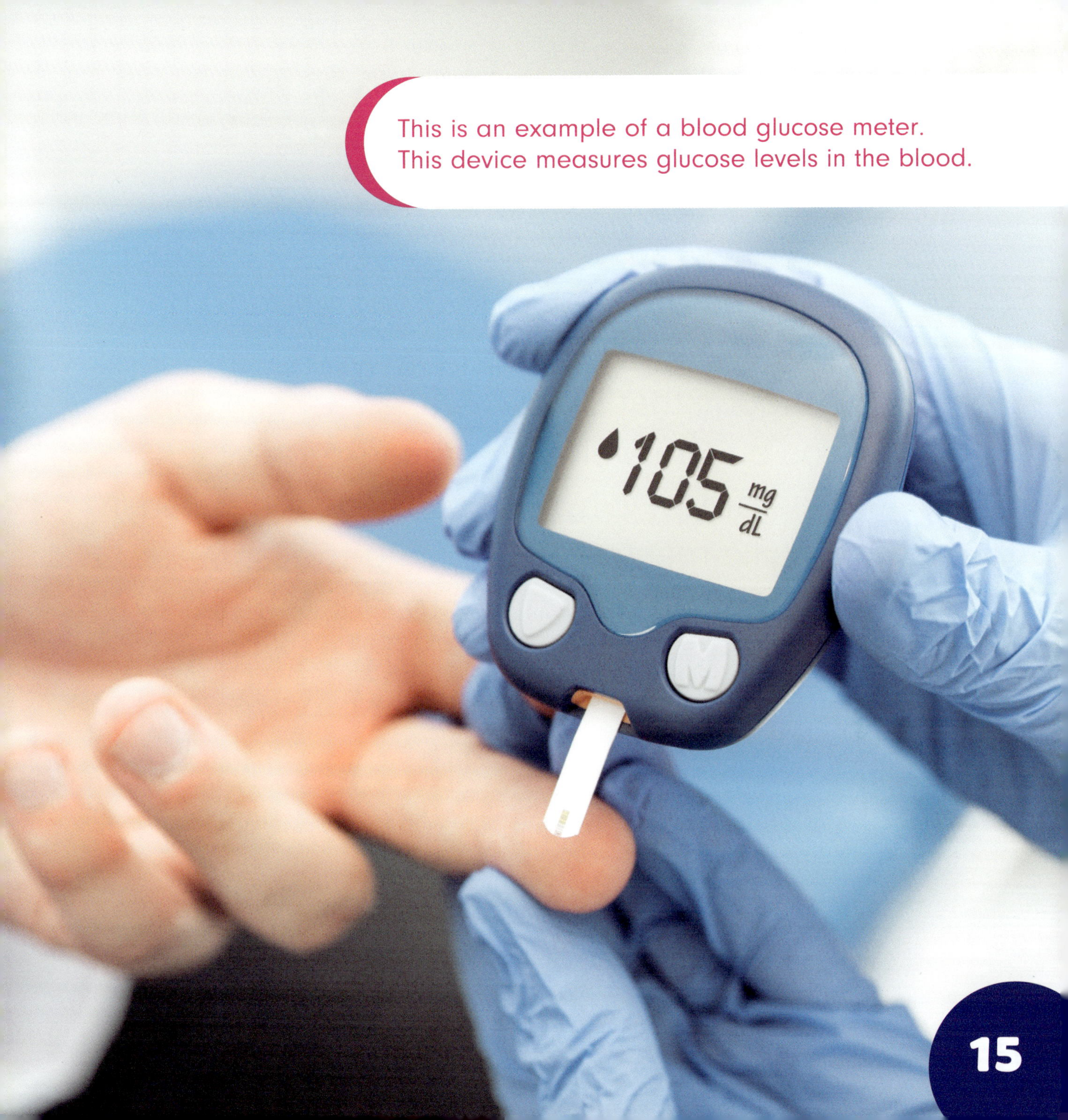

This is an example of a blood glucose meter. This device measures glucose levels in the blood.

On the Menu

Do you have to give up your favorite foods if you have diabetes? No! But you do need to be smart about what you eat and when.

Even foods that don't taste sweet can cause high blood sugar levels. This can include white rice and potatoes. Why? These foods are called starches. Like many sweet-tasting foods, the body breaks down starches into glucose.

A **dietician** can help you understand how different foods fit your care plan. Some foods, such as ice cream, may require an insulin dose before they're eaten.

Your Point of View

Many people match their insulin dose to the number of **carbohydrates** in their meal.

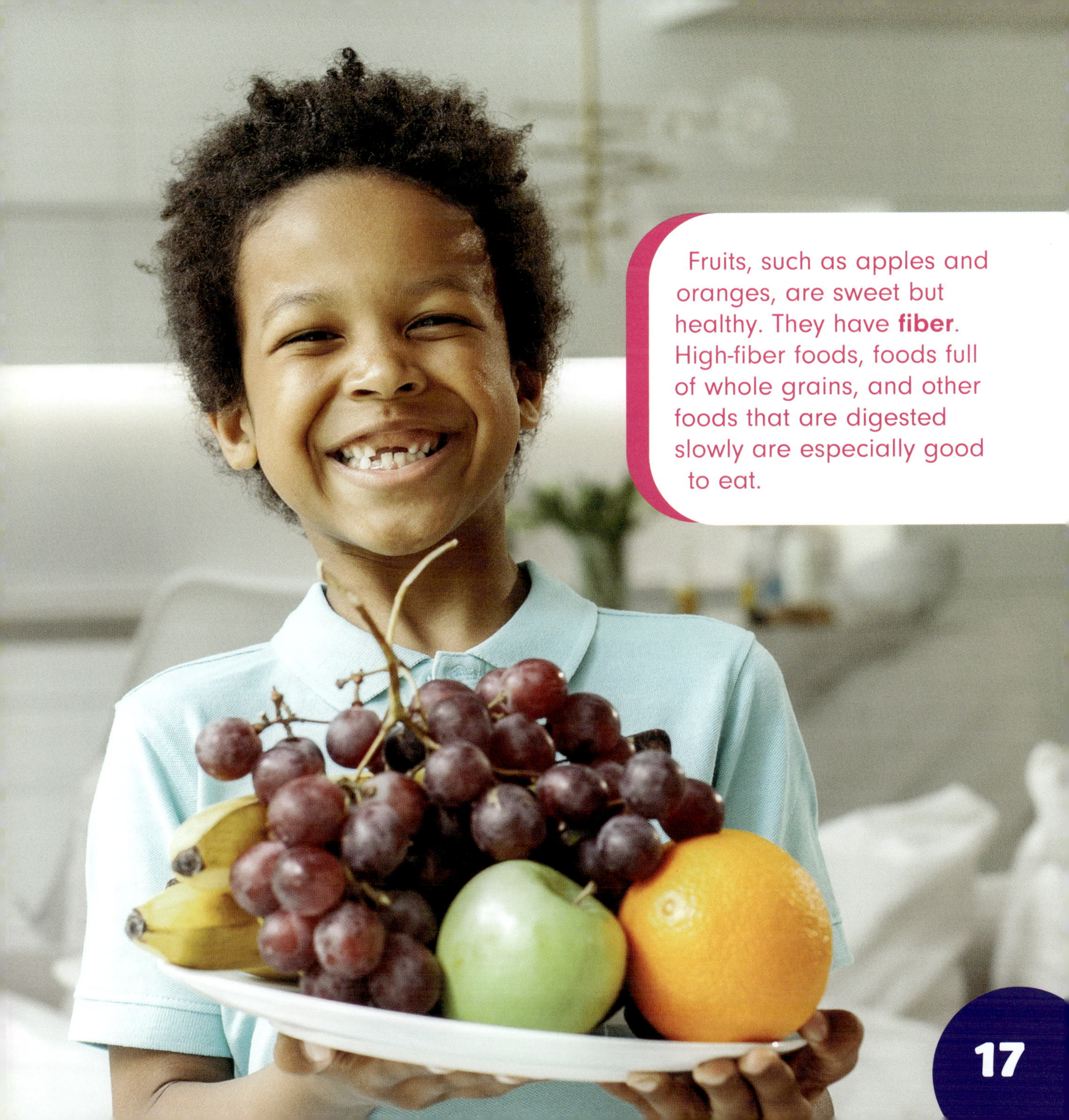

Fruits, such as apples and oranges, are sweet but healthy. They have **fiber**. High-fiber foods, foods full of whole grains, and other foods that are digested slowly are especially good to eat.

Dealing With Diabetes

A diabetes treatment plan will likely seem like a lot to learn at first. It may feel **overwhelming**. That's normal. You'll have a lot of help from trusted adults. These may include teachers, coaches, school nurses, and others who look out for you when your family can't be there.

But you should also learn how to care for yourself. It will get easier over time. And when you make a life change, such as joining a sports team, monitor your blood sugar levels more closely for a while.

When kids learn they have diabetes, they have a lot of feelings, such as anger, sadness, or fear. That's OK! It's important to talk to trusted adults about your feelings.

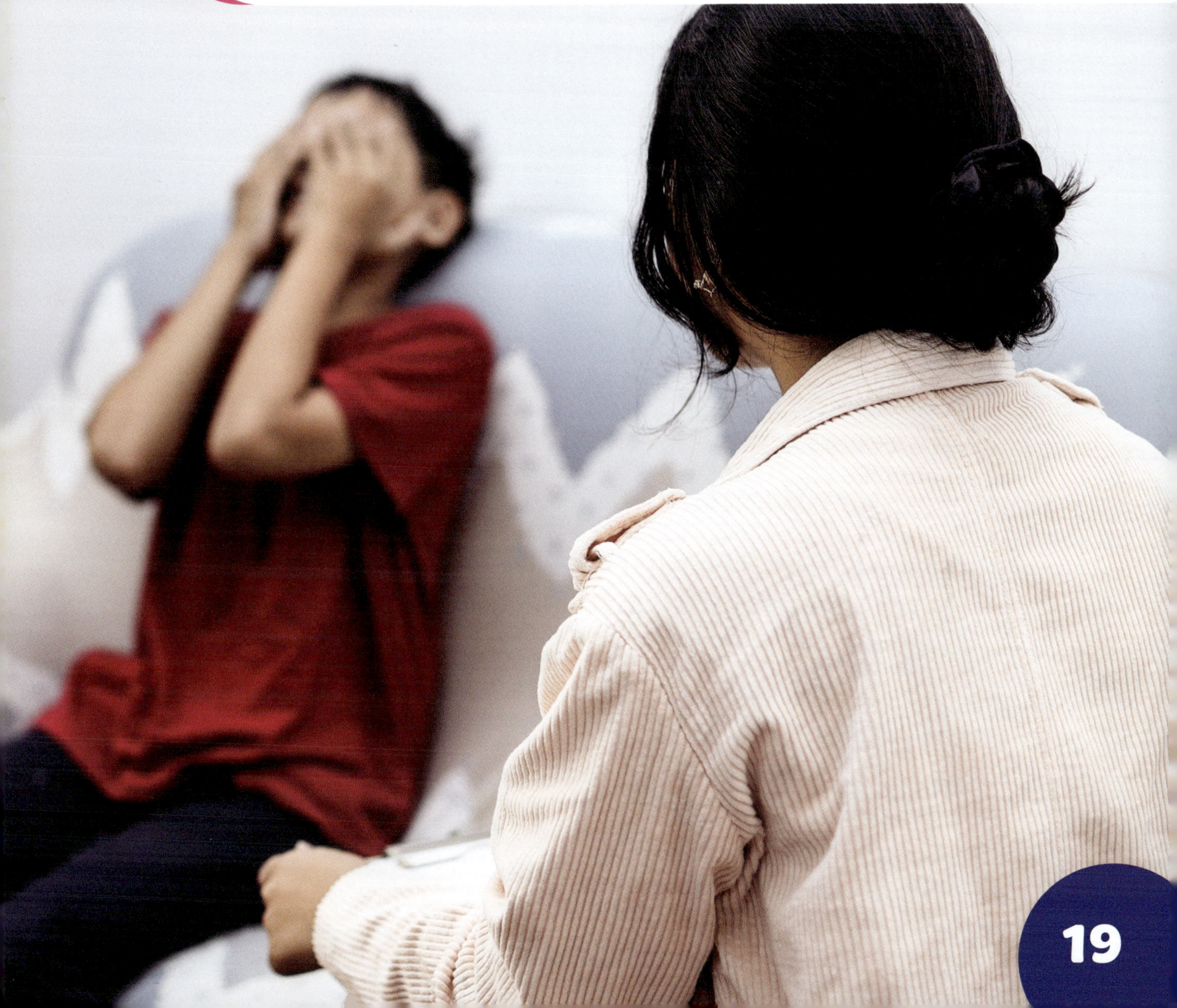

Friends Can Help

You'll learn to fit diabetes care into your life. That means not keeping it secret. Talk to your close friends about it when you're ready. They'll be curious what diabetes is, how it affects you, and how you care for yourself. If you feel shy, your parents and your friends' parents can help you explain.

You can't control if you have diabetes. You can control how you care for yourself. That means following your plan, telling people if it's not working, and getting back to being a kid!

Your Point of View

Scientists are always working on treatments to make living with diabetes easier. They haven't yet figured out why people get type 1 diabetes. It might in people's **genes**.

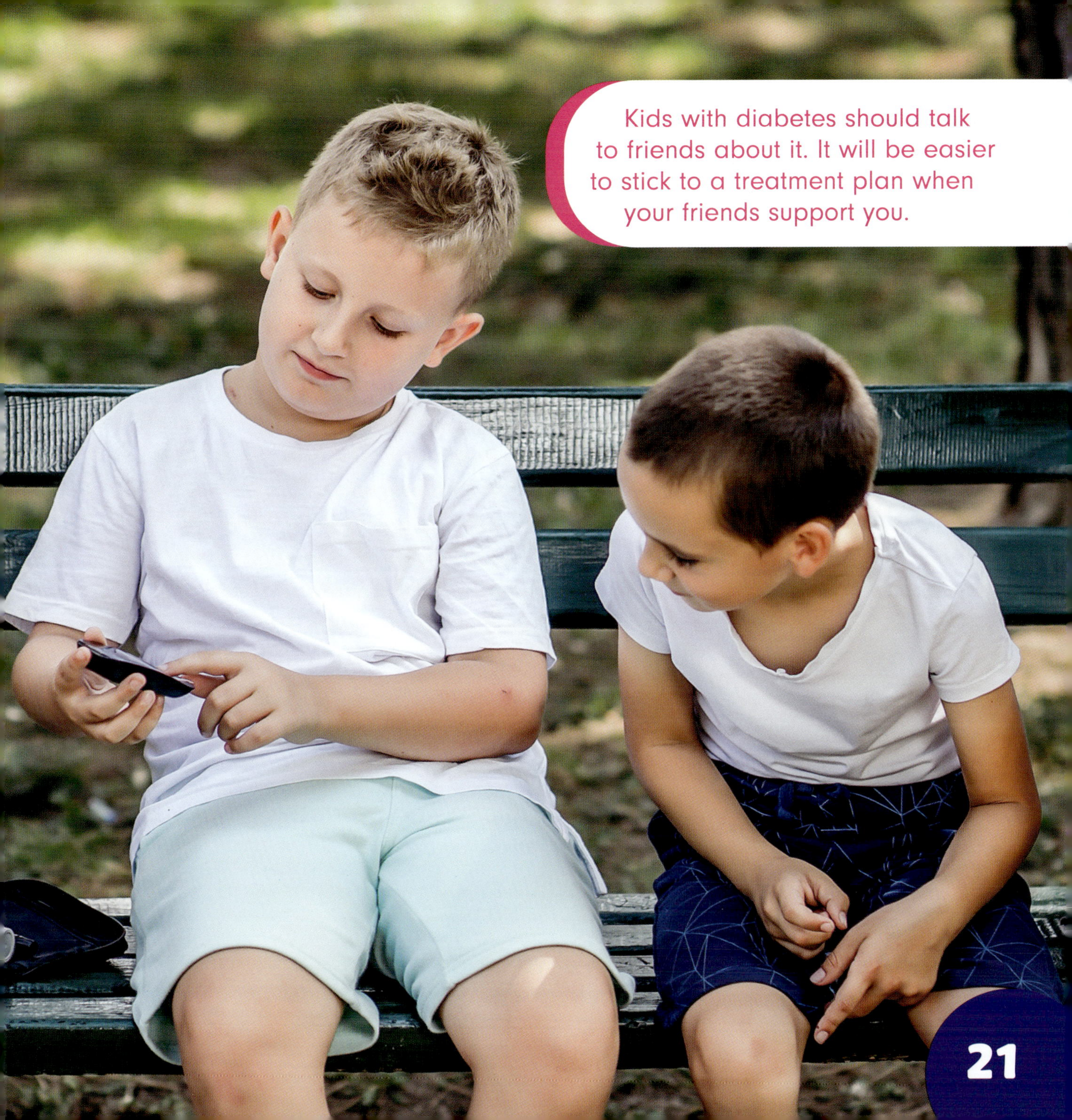

Kids with diabetes should talk to friends about it. It will be easier to stick to a treatment plan when your friends support you.

Glossary

acid: A liquid that breaks down matter.

blood vessel: A small tube in the body that carries blood.

carbohydrate: A nutrient in food that the body uses for energy. Sugars and starches are carbohydrates.

dietician: One whose job is to give people advice about what to eat.

fiber: Plant matter that can't be digested but helps digest other food.

gene: A tiny part of a cell that's passed along from parent to child and that decides specific features in the child, such as eye color.

hormone: A chemical made in the body that tells another part of the body what to do.

nerve: A part of the body that sends messages to the brain and allows someone to feel things.

overwhelming: A feeling that you can't do something because it seems so confusing or hard.

reaction: The way the body is affected by a drug or food, often badly.

symptom: A sign that shows someone is sick or has a certain condition.

For More Information

Books

Carser, A. R. *Handling Diabetes*. Minneapolis, MN: Essential Library, 2022.

Dickmann, Nancy. *Living with Diabetes.* Tucson, AZ: Brown Bear Books, 2023.

Schuh, Mari C. *My Life with Diabetes*. Mankato, MN: Amicus, 2024.

Websites

Diabetes Center
kidshealth.org/Advocate/en/kids/center/diabetes-center.html
This site is written for young people with diabetes.

Healthy Eating for Kids with Diabetes
kidshealth.org/en/kids/meal-plans-diabetes.html
Learn more about diabetes's connection to food.

Insulin and Monitoring Blood Sugar
childrens.dartmouth-health.org/diabetes-education/insulin-monitoring-blood-sugar
Find out about the different kinds of insulin.

Index